A NEW YOU! WORKOUT WORKBOOK

BY KYLA LATRICE, MBA

"IT'S TIME FOR YOU TO MOVE FROM
THE BACK OF THE LINE TO THE FRONT OF THE LINE"

A WORKBOOK FOR WOMEN AND MEN

A NEW YOU!
WORKOUT WORKBOOK

ALSO BY KYLA LATRICE, MBA

"New Me, New You! (How I Overcame Obesity)"

"The 7 Day Smoothie Detox"

"The 21 Day Slushie & Juice Fast"

"The 21 Day Salad Fast"

"Eat Well and Stay Thin (Living a Healthy You)"

"21 Days to a New Healthy You! Hearty Vegan & Vegetarian Slow Cooker Recipes"

"Twenty-One Healthy Ice Pop Snack Recipes"

"21 Days of Everyday Healthy Snack Recipes"

"All Natural Soups & Stews"

"A Collection of My Favorite Health Recipes"

A NEW YOU!
WORKOUT WORKBOOK

AN EXERCISE WORKOUT WORKBOOK TO PLAN YOUR WORKOUTS SO THAT YOU CAN BECOME HEALTHY AND FIT OVER THE NEXT 21 DAYS WITH A ONE MONTH, THREE MONTH AND SIX MONTH UPDATE FOR A TOTAL OF 63 DAYS

BONUS: AN EXTRA 2 DAYS OF WORKOUT PLAN SCHEDULES HAVE BEEN ADDED TO THE WORKBOOK

KYLA LATRICE, MBA

Lady Mirage Publications, Inc.

New York   Memphis   Los Angeles   London   Cape Town   Toronto
Atlanta   Singapore   Japan

Copyright © 2014 by Ms. Kyla Latrice, Inc.
The author is represented by Lady Mirage Literary Agency, Inc.
All rights reserved. In accordance with the U.S. Copyright Act of 1976, the scanning, uploading, and electronic sharing of any part of this book without the permission of the publisher is unlawful piracy and theft of the author's intellectual property. If you would like to use material from the book (other than for review purposes), prior written permission must be obtained by contacting the publisher at www.LadyMirageAgency.com
Thank you for your support of the author's rights.

Published by:
Lady Mirage Publications, Inc.
3724 Goodman Rd W, Unit 575
Horn Lake, MS 38637
www.LadyMirageAgency.com

Manufactured in the United States of America
First Edition: June 2014

Lady Mirage Publications, Inc. is an imprint and subsidiary
of Lady Mirage Global. The Lady Mirage Publications, Inc. name and logo are trademarks of
Lady Mirage Global.

Authors within the Lady Mirage Global (under Lady Mirage Agency, Inc.), Lady Mirage Publications and Lady Mirage Literary Agency speakers division provides a wide range of authors for speaking engagements.
To find out more information, go to www.LadyMirageAgency.com

The publisher is not responsible for websites (or their content) that are not owned by the publisher.

eISBN: 978-1-31-080226-3; Print ISBN: 978-0-9975371-4-7

Tennin, Kyla Latrice.
   A New You! Workout Workbook
      Pages cm; copyrighted materials.

Print Edition, License Note

This Workbook is licensed for your personal enjoyment only. This Workbook may not be re-sold or given away to other people. If you would like to share this Workbook with another person, please purchase an additional copy for each recipient. If you're reading this Workbook and did not purchase it, or it was not purchased for your use only, then please return to your favorite Bookseller or Retailer and purchase your own copy. Thank you for respecting the hard work of this author.

Also Note

In this Workbook, Ms. Latrice begins by explaining ***fitness plans*** that she has created, tested and tried, which significantly contributed to her weight loss, weight management and healthy eating lifestyle journey.
She has also written this Workbook due to there being so many books, DVDs and health, weight loss, fitness and "diet" programs currently being on the global market. The programs and books she has seen and reviewed are too long, too thick, have too much information and many times, are difficult for people to read. This Workbook was written to ***simplify and shorten*** how to lose weight and maintain your health, for life. It is based on personal experience and is still done today. It's an effective solution.

TABLE OF CONTENTS

Also By Kyla Latrice, MBA..2
   Copyright Page...4
      Purpose of Workbook...7
A New Healthy You: 5 Reasons..9
   A New Healthy You: Fitness Plan..10
      A New Healthy You: Workout Schedule Sample......................................11
A New Healthy You: Fitness Examples..12
   A New Healthy You: Nutrition Lifestyle Evaluation: Month ONE......................13
A New Healthy You: Nutrition Lifestyle Evaluation: Month THREE..................................14
   A New Healthy You: Nutrition Lifestyle Evaluation: Month SIX.........................15
A New Healthy You: Workout Schedule Day 1-65...16-80
Congratulations on the New You!...82

PURPOSE

Someone once said, when you don't know *the purpose of a thing* you will abuse it. Here is the purpose of this manual, so you can begin your NEW YOU the right way, *from the beginning.*

The purpose of this workout workbook is to assist you with starting over, better this time, with a fresh start on your health. To help you jumpstart the new you I have enclosed some work out tips and tricks.

In addition, to make your workouts and journey to becoming healthier, *easier*, in today's busy society, I have made this workbook available for people that are mobile, whom travel, work long hours, have many errands to run, are busy moms, busy dads or just don't have a lot of time to commit to long exercise routines or gym memberships.
You're "on-the-go".

"ON-THE-GO" This workbook *(and all of my cookbooks, books, workbooks and manuals)* can be read and applied in airports, on trains, at work on your lunch break, in the grocery store while shopping for and planning your weekly meals, at restaurants *(for quick decision making; to remember your health and/or weight loss goals),* in shopping malls, at fast food restaurants (to pull up and look at to remember your goals before ordering), at the park (before a jog), during your hotel stays, on vacations and at airport food counters when ordering your meals and beverages.

This workbook has been made available on mobile devices via Adobe Digital Editions and DRM (Digital Rights Management).

CONNECT WITH US
MAKING A DIFFERENCE IN THE LIVES OF MILLIONS, AROUND THE WORLD
Connect via Facebook Fan Page, YouTube and others by typing in **KYLA LATRICE MBA**

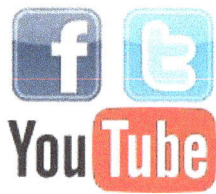

A NEW YOU!
WORKOUT WORKBOOK

A NEW HEALTHY YOU!
5 Reasons
"Why I Want To Get Healthy and Reach My Goal Weight" Assessment

Name: _____
Date: _____
Goal Weight: _____

  Before you begin compiling your list of reasons why you would like to get healthier and/or lose weight, ***think*** about your reasons first. It is crucial that your reasons be personal and not to please others. So, be specific with your "top 5" choices.

  Take a few moments from each day to thoughtfully read through your list to program your reasons in your mind. If you find it more convenient you can even transfer your list to a 3x5 index card to keep in your purse or wallet, one in your office at work, one in your car (for those fast food restaurant stops) and even one on your refrigerator at home (to think about what you're eating "before" you eat).

  Make a commitment to yourself now and state aloud: "I will read my health index card whenever I am confronted with a difficult food situation." Reading this list will help you reinforce your personal commitment to taking control of your health ***and*** weight instead of them taking control over you.

1. _____

2. _____

3. _____

4. _____

5. _____

A NEW HEALTHY YOU!
Fitness Plan

DAILY WORKOUT PLAN
To complete the exercise worksheet schedule as a tracker of your fitness goals progress, place a check mark or "x" in the completed (x) section when you have completed your "No Workout" and "Workout" scheduled times.

NON-WORKOUT DAYS
On your **"Non-Workout Days"** you will do the following: 100 crunches before bedtime (2 sets, 50 each), standing leg lifts (2 sets, one set for each leg, 10-18 repetitions) and light stretching (arms and legs as you feel necessary). Stretching can be while standing or sitting and toe touches. Your Non-workout days can be done once or twice a week, to keep your metabolism regular, to speed it up as well as to work on flattening and toning your midsection *(stomach)*.

WORKOUT DAYS
On your **"Workout Days"** you will do the workout <u>plan</u> below. Stretching can be while standing or sitting and toe touches. Your workout days should be done 3-4 times a week, to speed up your metabolism as well as to work on losing weight, creating a stable weight once you reach your goal and toning.

- Standing leg lifts (2 sets, one set for each leg, 10-18 repetitions)
- Standing front leg lifts (2 sets, one set for each leg, 10-18 repetitions)
- Standing back leg lifts (2 sets, one set for each leg, 10-18 repetitions)
- Standing side leg lifts (2 sets, one set for each leg, 10-18 repetitions)
- Arm circles (front) (2 sets, 25 repetitions)
- Arm circles (back) (2 sets, 25 repetitions)
- Squats (2 sets, 10 repetitions)
- Arm Stretching (forearms and back arms) (1 set each, for each arm, hold for 10 seconds each)
- Light stretching (Toe Touches; Standing and Sitting; Front of Leg and Side of Leg Stretching)
- Side leg lifts (laying down) (2 sets, one for each leg, 10-25 repetitions)
- 100 crunches (50 Frontwards and 25 on the Right Side Ab and 25 on the Left Side Ab)
- Leg rotations in the air (bicycling; frontwards and backwards) (1 set, 25 each)
- Leg scissors in the air (1 set, 10-15 each)
- Leg raises in the air (1 set, 10-15 each)
- Leg separations in the air (1 set, 10-15 each)

And again…

- Leg rotations in the air (bicycling; frontwards and backwards) (1 set, 25 each)
- Leg scissors in the air (1 set, 10-15 each)
- Leg raises in the air (1 set, 10-15 each)
- Leg separations in the air (1 set, 10-15 each)

Then…

- Back of Leg lifts (2 sets, 25 each)
- Back of Leg, Rainbows on one knee and one elbow (make a rainbow) (1 set, 10-15 per leg)

A NEW HEALTHY YOU!
Workout Plan Schedule

SAMPLE

*Saturdays – Weight yourself at 7am and record the weight to keep track of your progress.

Date	Week	Day	Exercise	Completed (x)	Weigh In	Workout Time
	1	Monday	No workout			
		Tuesday	Workout	x		30 minutes (Lightly)
		Wednesday	No workout			
		Thursday	Workout	x		30 minutes (Lightly)
		Friday	No workout			
		Saturday*	Workout	x	234	30 minutes (Lightly)
		Sunday	No workout			
	2	Monday	Workout	x		30 minutes (Lightly)
		Tuesday	No workout			
		Wednesday	Workout			30 minutes (Lightly)
		Thursday	No workout			
		Friday	Workout	x		30 minutes (Lightly)
		Saturday*	No workout		211	
		Sunday	Workout			30 minutes (Lightly)
	3	Monday	No workout			
		Tuesday	Workout	x		30 minutes (Lightly)
		Wednesday	No workout			
		Thursday	Workout	x		30 minutes (Lightly)
		Friday	No workout			
		Saturday*	Workout		196	30 minutes (Lightly)
		Sunday	No workout			

A NEW HEALTHY YOU!
Fitness Examples

Stretching [Toe Touches; Both Sides]

Stretching [Toe Touches; Front]

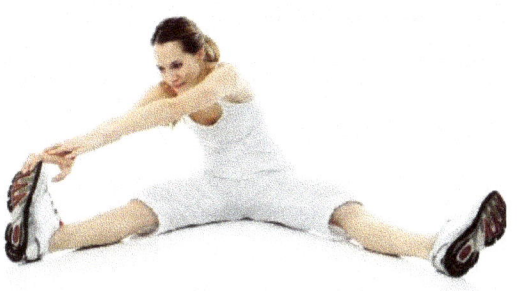
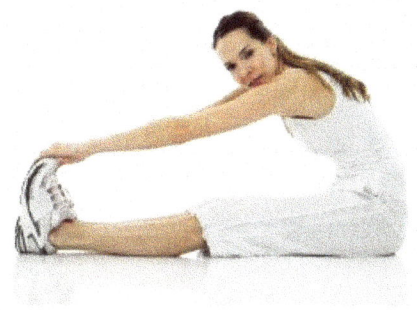

Arm Circles [Frontwards & Backwards]

Front of Leg Stretching [Front of Each Leg]

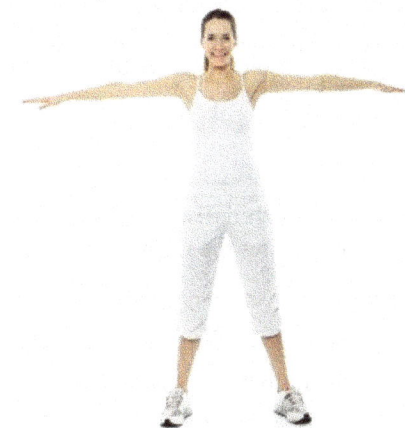
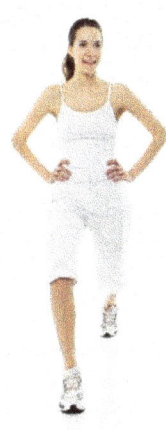

Back of Leg Lifts [Right & Left Leg]

Crunches [Frontwards & Sidewards]

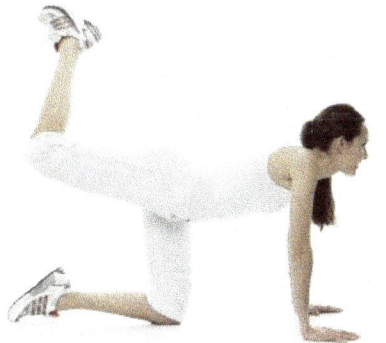
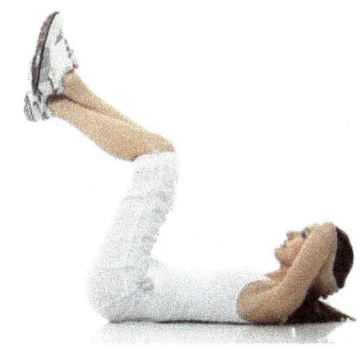

Photo Credits: Ambro; FreeDigitalPhotos.net

A NEW HEALTHY YOU!
Nutrition, Health and Lifestyle Evaluation
MONTH ONE
Please Record Your Information for the First Month of Working on Your "New You"

Current Weight: _____

Name: _____

Date: _____

1. What is your main reason for wanting to lose weight? _____
2. What is your weight goal? _____
3. When did you begin gaining excess weight? (give reasons, if known) _____
4. What is the most you have weighed (non-pregnant) and when? _____
5. Are any of your family members overweight? (circle one)   Yes   No
6. How often per week do you eat out? _____ Times per week you eat "fast food?" _____
7. Weight at 18-25 years old? _____ Weight one year ago? _____
8. Foods you crave: _____
9. Do you drink coffee, sodas or tea? Yes   No   How much daily? _____
10. Do you wake up hungry first thing in the morning or during the night? Yes No If, yes, how often? _____
11. Previous diets you have tried and your results: _____
12. How often do you work out? (circle one)   Never   Occasionally   Several Times a Week
13. Do you drink alcohol (circle one)?   No   Occasionally   Weekly   Daily
If yes, circle all that you drink   Beer   Wine   Distilled Spirits   Other
14. Smoking Habits (choose only one)

_____ You have never smoked cigarettes, cigars or a pipe

_____ You have quit smoking ____ years ago and have not smoked since
If so, how long did you smoke before you quit?

_____ You smoke: How many packs per day _____

Note: Any physical activity can be considered as a workout, such as golf, tennis, jogging, swimming, cycling, etc.

A NEW HEALTHY YOU!
Nutrition, Health and Lifestyle Evaluation
MONTH THREE
Please Record Your Information for the Third Month of Working on Your "New You"

Current Weight: _____

Name: _____

Date: _____

1. What is your main reason for wanting to lose weight? _____
2. What is your weight goal? _____
3. When did you begin gaining excess weight? (give reasons, if known) _____
4. What is the most you have weighed (non-pregnant) and when? _____
5. Are any of your family members overweight? (circle one)   Yes   No
6. How often per week do you eat out? _____ Times per week you eat "fast food?" _____
7. Weight at 18-25 years old? _____ Weight one year ago? _____
8. Foods you crave: _____
9. Do you drink coffee, sodas or tea? Yes   No   How much daily? _____
10. Do you wake up hungry first thing in the morning or during the night? Yes No If, yes, how often? _____
11. Previous diets you have tried and your results: _____
12. How often do you work out? (circle one)   Never   Occasionally   Several Times a Week
13. Do you drink alcohol (circle one)?   No   Occasionally   Weekly   Daily
    If yes, circle all that you drink   Beer   Wine   Distilled Spirits   Other
14. Smoking Habits   (choose only one)

    _____ You have never smoked cigarettes, cigars or a pipe

    _____ You have quit smoking _____ years ago and have not smoked since
    If so, how long did you smoke before you quit?

    _____ You smoke: How many packs per day _____

Note: Any physical activity can be considered as a workout, such as golf, tennis, jogging, swimming, cycling, etc.

A NEW HEALTHY YOU!
Nutrition, Health and Lifestyle Evaluation
MONTH SIX
Please Record Your Information for the Sixth Month of Working on Your "New You"

Current Weight: _____

Name: _____

Date: _____

1. What is your main reason for wanting to lose weight? _____
2. What is your weight goal? _____
3. When did you begin gaining excess weight? (give reasons, if known) _____
4. What is the most you have weighed (non-pregnant) and when? _____
5. Are any of your family members overweight? (circle one)   Yes   No
6. How often per week do you eat out? _____ Times per week you eat "fast food?" _____
7. Weight at 18-25 years old? _____ Weight one year ago? _____
8. Foods you crave: _____
9. Do you drink coffee, sodas or tea? Yes   No   How much daily? _____
10. Do you wake up hungry first thing in the morning or during the night? Yes No If, yes, how often? _____
11. Previous diets you have tried and your results: _____
12. How often do you work out? (circle one)   Never   Occasionally   Several Times a Week
13. Do you drink alcohol (circle one)?   No   Occasionally   Weekly   Daily
    If yes, circle all that you drink   Beer   Wine   Distilled Spirits   Other
14. Smoking Habits   (choose only one)

    _____ You have never smoked cigarettes, cigars or a pipe

    _____ You have quit smoking ____ years ago and have not smoked since
    If so, how long did you smoke before you quit?

    _____ You smoke: How many packs per day _____

Note: Any physical activity can be considered as a workout, such as golf, tennis, jogging, swimming, cycling, etc.

A NEW HEALTHY YOU!
Workout Plan Schedule

DAY 1

Date	Week	Day	Exercise	Completed (x)	Weigh In	Workout Time
	1	Monday	No workout			
		Tuesday	Workout			30 minutes (Lightly)
		Wednesday	No workout			
		Thursday	Workout			30 minutes (Lightly)
		Friday	No workout			
		Saturday*	Workout			30 minutes (Lightly)
		Sunday	No workout			
	2	Monday	Workout			30 minutes (Lightly)
		Tuesday	No workout			
		Wednesday	Workout			30 minutes (Lightly)
		Thursday	No workout			
		Friday	Workout			30 minutes (Lightly)
		Saturday*	No workout			
		Sunday	Workout			30 minutes (Lightly)
	3	Monday	No workout			
		Tuesday	Workout			30 minutes (Lightly)
		Wednesday	No workout			
		Thursday	Workout			30 minutes (Lightly)
		Friday	No workout			
		Saturday*	Workout			30 minutes (Lightly)
		Sunday	No workout			

A NEW HEALTHY YOU!
Workout Plan Schedule

DAY 2

Date	Week	Day	Exercise	Completed (x)	Weigh In	Workout Time
	1	Monday	No workout			
		Tuesday	Workout			30 minutes (Lightly)
		Wednesday	No workout			
		Thursday	Workout			30 minutes (Lightly)
		Friday	No workout			
		Saturday*	Workout			30 minutes (Lightly)
		Sunday	No workout			
	2	Monday	Workout			30 minutes (Lightly)
		Tuesday	No workout			
		Wednesday	Workout			30 minutes (Lightly)
		Thursday	No workout			
		Friday	Workout			30 minutes (Lightly)
		Saturday*	No workout			
		Sunday	Workout			30 minutes (Lightly)
	3	Monday	No workout			
		Tuesday	Workout			30 minutes (Lightly)
		Wednesday	No workout			
		Thursday	Workout			30 minutes (Lightly)
		Friday	No workout			
		Saturday*	Workout			30 minutes (Lightly)
		Sunday	No workout			

A NEW HEALTHY YOU!
Workout Plan Schedule

DAY 3

Date	Week	Day	Exercise	Completed (x)	Weigh In	Workout Time
	1	Monday	No workout			
		Tuesday	Workout			30 minutes (Lightly)
		Wednesday	No workout			
		Thursday	Workout			30 minutes (Lightly)
		Friday	No workout			
		Saturday*	Workout			30 minutes (Lightly)
		Sunday	No workout			
	2	Monday	Workout			30 minutes (Lightly)
		Tuesday	No workout			
		Wednesday	Workout			30 minutes (Lightly)
		Thursday	No workout			
		Friday	Workout			30 minutes (Lightly)
		Saturday*	No workout			
		Sunday	Workout			30 minutes (Lightly)
	3	Monday	No workout			
		Tuesday	Workout			30 minutes (Lightly)
		Wednesday	No workout			
		Thursday	Workout			30 minutes (Lightly)
		Friday	No workout			
		Saturday*	Workout			30 minutes (Lightly)
		Sunday	No workout			

A NEW HEALTHY YOU!
Workout Plan Schedule

DAY 4

Date	Week	Day	Exercise	Completed (x)	Weigh In	Workout Time
	1	Monday	No workout			
		Tuesday	Workout			30 minutes (Lightly)
		Wednesday	No workout			
		Thursday	Workout			30 minutes (Lightly)
		Friday	No workout			
		Saturday*	Workout			30 minutes (Lightly)
		Sunday	No workout			
	2	Monday	Workout			30 minutes (Lightly)
		Tuesday	No workout			
		Wednesday	Workout			30 minutes (Lightly)
		Thursday	No workout			
		Friday	Workout			30 minutes (Lightly)
		Saturday*	No workout			
		Sunday	Workout			30 minutes (Lightly)
	3	Monday	No workout			
		Tuesday	Workout			30 minutes (Lightly)
		Wednesday	No workout			
		Thursday	Workout			30 minutes (Lightly)
		Friday	No workout			
		Saturday*	Workout			30 minutes (Lightly)
		Sunday	No workout			

A NEW HEALTHY YOU!
Workout Plan Schedule

DAY 5

Date	Week	Day	Exercise	Completed (x)	Weigh In	Workout Time
	1	Monday	No workout			
		Tuesday	Workout			30 minutes (Lightly)
		Wednesday	No workout			
		Thursday	Workout			30 minutes (Lightly)
		Friday	No workout			
		Saturday*	Workout			30 minutes (Lightly)
		Sunday	No workout			
	2	Monday	Workout			30 minutes (Lightly)
		Tuesday	No workout			
		Wednesday	Workout			30 minutes (Lightly)
		Thursday	No workout			
		Friday	Workout			30 minutes (Lightly)
		Saturday*	No workout			
		Sunday	Workout			30 minutes (Lightly)
	3	Monday	No workout			
		Tuesday	Workout			30 minutes (Lightly)
		Wednesday	No workout			
		Thursday	Workout			30 minutes (Lightly)
		Friday	No workout			
		Saturday*	Workout			30 minutes (Lightly)
		Sunday	No workout			

A NEW HEALTHY YOU!
Workout Plan Schedule

DAY 6

Date	Week	Day	Exercise	Completed (x)	Weigh In	Workout Time
	1	Monday	No workout			
		Tuesday	Workout			30 minutes (Lightly)
		Wednesday	No workout			
		Thursday	Workout			30 minutes (Lightly)
		Friday	No workout			
		Saturday*	Workout			30 minutes (Lightly)
		Sunday	No workout			
	2	Monday	Workout			30 minutes (Lightly)
		Tuesday	No workout			
		Wednesday	Workout			30 minutes (Lightly)
		Thursday	No workout			
		Friday	Workout			30 minutes (Lightly)
		Saturday*	No workout			
		Sunday	Workout			30 minutes (Lightly)
	3	Monday	No workout			
		Tuesday	Workout			30 minutes (Lightly)
		Wednesday	No workout			
		Thursday	Workout			30 minutes (Lightly)
		Friday	No workout			
		Saturday*	Workout			30 minutes (Lightly)
		Sunday	No workout			

A NEW HEALTHY YOU!
Workout Plan Schedule

DAY 7

Date	Week	Day	Exercise	Completed (x)	Weigh In	Workout Time
	1	Monday	No workout			
		Tuesday	Workout			30 minutes (Lightly)
		Wednesday	No workout			
		Thursday	Workout			30 minutes (Lightly)
		Friday	No workout			
		Saturday*	Workout			30 minutes (Lightly)
		Sunday	No workout			
	2	Monday	Workout			30 minutes (Lightly)
		Tuesday	No workout			
		Wednesday	Workout			30 minutes (Lightly)
		Thursday	No workout			
		Friday	Workout			30 minutes (Lightly)
		Saturday*	No workout			
		Sunday	Workout			30 minutes (Lightly)
	3	Monday	No workout			
		Tuesday	Workout			30 minutes (Lightly)
		Wednesday	No workout			
		Thursday	Workout			30 minutes (Lightly)
		Friday	No workout			
		Saturday*	Workout			30 minutes (Lightly)
		Sunday	No workout			

A NEW HEALTHY YOU!
Workout Plan Schedule

DAY 8

Date	Week	Day	Exercise	Completed (x)	Weigh In	Workout Time
	1	Monday	No workout			
		Tuesday	Workout			30 minutes (Lightly)
		Wednesday	No workout			
		Thursday	Workout			30 minutes (Lightly)
		Friday	No workout			
		Saturday*	Workout			30 minutes (Lightly)
		Sunday	No workout			
	2	Monday	Workout			30 minutes (Lightly)
		Tuesday	No workout			
		Wednesday	Workout			30 minutes (Lightly)
		Thursday	No workout			
		Friday	Workout			30 minutes (Lightly)
		Saturday*	No workout			
		Sunday	Workout			30 minutes (Lightly)
	3	Monday	No workout			
		Tuesday	Workout			30 minutes (Lightly)
		Wednesday	No workout			
		Thursday	Workout			30 minutes (Lightly)
		Friday	No workout			
		Saturday*	Workout			30 minutes (Lightly)
		Sunday	No workout			

A NEW HEALTHY YOU!
Workout Plan Schedule

DAY 9

Date	Week	Day	Exercise	Completed (x)	Weigh In	Workout Time
	1	Monday	No workout			
		Tuesday	Workout			30 minutes (Lightly)
		Wednesday	No workout			
		Thursday	Workout			30 minutes (Lightly)
		Friday	No workout			
		Saturday*	Workout			30 minutes (Lightly)
		Sunday	No workout			
	2	Monday	Workout			30 minutes (Lightly)
		Tuesday	No workout			
		Wednesday	Workout			30 minutes (Lightly)
		Thursday	No workout			
		Friday	Workout			30 minutes (Lightly)
		Saturday*	No workout			
		Sunday	Workout			30 minutes (Lightly)
	3	Monday	No workout			
		Tuesday	Workout			30 minutes (Lightly)
		Wednesday	No workout			
		Thursday	Workout			30 minutes (Lightly)
		Friday	No workout			
		Saturday*	Workout			30 minutes (Lightly)
		Sunday	No workout			

A NEW HEALTHY YOU!
Workout Plan Schedule

DAY 10

Date	Week	Day	Exercise	Completed (x)	Weigh In	Workout Time
	1	Monday	No workout			
		Tuesday	Workout			30 minutes (Lightly)
		Wednesday	No workout			
		Thursday	Workout			30 minutes (Lightly)
		Friday	No workout			
		Saturday*	Workout			30 minutes (Lightly)
		Sunday	No workout			
	2	Monday	Workout			30 minutes (Lightly)
		Tuesday	No workout			
		Wednesday	Workout			30 minutes (Lightly)
		Thursday	No workout			
		Friday	Workout			30 minutes (Lightly)
		Saturday*	No workout			
		Sunday	Workout			30 minutes (Lightly)
	3	Monday	No workout			
		Tuesday	Workout			30 minutes (Lightly)
		Wednesday	No workout			
		Thursday	Workout			30 minutes (Lightly)
		Friday	No workout			
		Saturday*	Workout			30 minutes (Lightly)
		Sunday	No workout			

A NEW HEALTHY YOU!
Workout Plan Schedule

DAY 11

Date	Week	Day	Exercise	Completed (x)	Weigh In	Workout Time
	1	Monday	No workout			
		Tuesday	Workout			30 minutes (Lightly)
		Wednesday	No workout			
		Thursday	Workout			30 minutes (Lightly)
		Friday	No workout			
		Saturday*	Workout			30 minutes (Lightly)
		Sunday	No workout			
	2	Monday	Workout			30 minutes (Lightly)
		Tuesday	No workout			
		Wednesday	Workout			30 minutes (Lightly)
		Thursday	No workout			
		Friday	Workout			30 minutes (Lightly)
		Saturday*	No workout			
		Sunday	Workout			30 minutes (Lightly)
	3	Monday	No workout			
		Tuesday	Workout			30 minutes (Lightly)
		Wednesday	No workout			
		Thursday	Workout			30 minutes (Lightly)
		Friday	No workout			
		Saturday*	Workout			30 minutes (Lightly)
		Sunday	No workout			

A NEW HEALTHY YOU!
Workout Plan Schedule

DAY 12

Date	Week	Day	Exercise	Completed (x)	Weigh In	Workout Time
	1	Monday	No workout			
		Tuesday	Workout			30 minutes (Lightly)
		Wednesday	No workout			
		Thursday	Workout			30 minutes (Lightly)
		Friday	No workout			
		Saturday*	Workout			30 minutes (Lightly)
		Sunday	No workout			
	2	Monday	Workout			30 minutes (Lightly)
		Tuesday	No workout			
		Wednesday	Workout			30 minutes (Lightly)
		Thursday	No workout			
		Friday	Workout			30 minutes (Lightly)
		Saturday*	No workout			
		Sunday	Workout			30 minutes (Lightly)
	3	Monday	No workout			
		Tuesday	Workout			30 minutes (Lightly)
		Wednesday	No workout			
		Thursday	Workout			30 minutes (Lightly)
		Friday	No workout			
		Saturday*	Workout			30 minutes (Lightly)
		Sunday	No workout			

A NEW HEALTHY YOU!
Workout Plan Schedule

DAY 13

Date	Week	Day	Exercise	Completed (x)	Weigh In	Workout Time
	1	Monday	No workout			
		Tuesday	Workout			30 minutes (Lightly)
		Wednesday	No workout			
		Thursday	Workout			30 minutes (Lightly)
		Friday	No workout			
		Saturday*	Workout			30 minutes (Lightly)
		Sunday	No workout			
	2	Monday	Workout			30 minutes (Lightly)
		Tuesday	No workout			
		Wednesday	Workout			30 minutes (Lightly)
		Thursday	No workout			
		Friday	Workout			30 minutes (Lightly)
		Saturday*	No workout			
		Sunday	Workout			30 minutes (Lightly)
	3	Monday	No workout			
		Tuesday	Workout			30 minutes (Lightly)
		Wednesday	No workout			
		Thursday	Workout			30 minutes (Lightly)
		Friday	No workout			
		Saturday*	Workout			30 minutes (Lightly)
		Sunday	No workout			

A NEW HEALTHY YOU!
Workout Plan Schedule

DAY 14

Date	Week	Day	Exercise	Completed (x)	Weigh In	Workout Time
	1	Monday	No workout			
		Tuesday	Workout			30 minutes (Lightly)
		Wednesday	No workout			
		Thursday	Workout			30 minutes (Lightly)
		Friday	No workout			
		Saturday*	Workout			30 minutes (Lightly)
		Sunday	No workout			
	2	Monday	Workout			30 minutes (Lightly)
		Tuesday	No workout			
		Wednesday	Workout			30 minutes (Lightly)
		Thursday	No workout			
		Friday	Workout			30 minutes (Lightly)
		Saturday*	No workout			
		Sunday	Workout			30 minutes (Lightly)
	3	Monday	No workout			
		Tuesday	Workout			30 minutes (Lightly)
		Wednesday	No workout			
		Thursday	Workout			30 minutes (Lightly)
		Friday	No workout			
		Saturday*	Workout			30 minutes (Lightly)
		Sunday	No workout			

A NEW HEALTHY YOU!
Workout Plan Schedule

DAY 15

Date	Week	Day	Exercise	Completed (x)	Weigh In	Workout Time
	1	Monday	No workout			
		Tuesday	Workout			30 minutes (Lightly)
		Wednesday	No workout			
		Thursday	Workout			30 minutes (Lightly)
		Friday	No workout			
		Saturday*	Workout			30 minutes (Lightly)
		Sunday	No workout			
	2	Monday	Workout			30 minutes (Lightly)
		Tuesday	No workout			
		Wednesday	Workout			30 minutes (Lightly)
		Thursday	No workout			
		Friday	Workout			30 minutes (Lightly)
		Saturday*	No workout			
		Sunday	Workout			30 minutes (Lightly)
	3	Monday	No workout			
		Tuesday	Workout			30 minutes (Lightly)
		Wednesday	No workout			
		Thursday	Workout			30 minutes (Lightly)
		Friday	No workout			
		Saturday*	Workout			30 minutes (Lightly)
		Sunday	No workout			

A NEW HEALTHY YOU!
Workout Plan Schedule

DAY 16

Date	Week	Day	Exercise	Completed (x)	Weigh In	Workout Time
	1	Monday	No workout			
		Tuesday	Workout			30 minutes (Lightly)
		Wednesday	No workout			
		Thursday	Workout			30 minutes (Lightly)
		Friday	No workout			
		Saturday*	Workout			30 minutes (Lightly)
		Sunday	No workout			
	2	Monday	Workout			30 minutes (Lightly)
		Tuesday	No workout			
		Wednesday	Workout			30 minutes (Lightly)
		Thursday	No workout			
		Friday	Workout			30 minutes (Lightly)
		Saturday*	No workout			
		Sunday	Workout			30 minutes (Lightly)
	3	Monday	No workout			
		Tuesday	Workout			30 minutes (Lightly)
		Wednesday	No workout			
		Thursday	Workout			30 minutes (Lightly)
		Friday	No workout			
		Saturday*	Workout			30 minutes (Lightly)
		Sunday	No workout			

A NEW HEALTHY YOU!
Workout Plan Schedule

DAY 17

Date	Week	Day	Exercise	Completed (x)	Weigh In	Workout Time
	1	Monday	No workout			
		Tuesday	Workout			30 minutes (Lightly)
		Wednesday	No workout			
		Thursday	Workout			30 minutes (Lightly)
		Friday	No workout			
		Saturday*	Workout			30 minutes (Lightly)
		Sunday	No workout			
	2	Monday	Workout			30 minutes (Lightly)
		Tuesday	No workout			
		Wednesday	Workout			30 minutes (Lightly)
		Thursday	No workout			
		Friday	Workout			30 minutes (Lightly)
		Saturday*	No workout			
		Sunday	Workout			30 minutes (Lightly)
	3	Monday	No workout			
		Tuesday	Workout			30 minutes (Lightly)
		Wednesday	No workout			
		Thursday	Workout			30 minutes (Lightly)
		Friday	No workout			
		Saturday*	Workout			30 minutes (Lightly)
		Sunday	No workout			

A NEW HEALTHY YOU!
Workout Plan Schedule

DAY 18

Date	Week	Day	Exercise	Completed (x)	Weigh In	Workout Time
	1	Monday	No workout			
		Tuesday	Workout			30 minutes (Lightly)
		Wednesday	No workout			
		Thursday	Workout			30 minutes (Lightly)
		Friday	No workout			
		Saturday*	Workout			30 minutes (Lightly)
		Sunday	No workout			
	2	Monday	Workout			30 minutes (Lightly)
		Tuesday	No workout			
		Wednesday	Workout			30 minutes (Lightly)
		Thursday	No workout			
		Friday	Workout			30 minutes (Lightly)
		Saturday*	No workout			
		Sunday	Workout			30 minutes (Lightly)
	3	Monday	No workout			
		Tuesday	Workout			30 minutes (Lightly)
		Wednesday	No workout			
		Thursday	Workout			30 minutes (Lightly)
		Friday	No workout			
		Saturday*	Workout			30 minutes (Lightly)
		Sunday	No workout			

A NEW HEALTHY YOU!
Workout Plan Schedule

DAY 19

Date	Week	Day	Exercise	Completed (x)	Weigh In	Workout Time
	1	Monday	No workout			
		Tuesday	Workout			30 minutes (Lightly)
		Wednesday	No workout			
		Thursday	Workout			30 minutes (Lightly)
		Friday	No workout			
		Saturday*	Workout			30 minutes (Lightly)
		Sunday	No workout			
	2	Monday	Workout			30 minutes (Lightly)
		Tuesday	No workout			
		Wednesday	Workout			30 minutes (Lightly)
		Thursday	No workout			
		Friday	Workout			30 minutes (Lightly)
		Saturday*	No workout			
		Sunday	Workout			30 minutes (Lightly)
	3	Monday	No workout			
		Tuesday	Workout			30 minutes (Lightly)
		Wednesday	No workout			
		Thursday	Workout			30 minutes (Lightly)
		Friday	No workout			
		Saturday*	Workout			30 minutes (Lightly)
		Sunday	No workout			

A NEW HEALTHY YOU!
Workout Plan Schedule

DAY 20

Date	Week	Day	Exercise	Completed (x)	Weigh In	Workout Time
	1	Monday	No workout			
		Tuesday	Workout			30 minutes (Lightly)
		Wednesday	No workout			
		Thursday	Workout			30 minutes (Lightly)
		Friday	No workout			
		Saturday*	Workout			30 minutes (Lightly)
		Sunday	No workout			
	2	Monday	Workout			30 minutes (Lightly)
		Tuesday	No workout			
		Wednesday	Workout			30 minutes (Lightly)
		Thursday	No workout			
		Friday	Workout			30 minutes (Lightly)
		Saturday*	No workout			
		Sunday	Workout			30 minutes (Lightly)
	3	Monday	No workout			
		Tuesday	Workout			30 minutes (Lightly)
		Wednesday	No workout			
		Thursday	Workout			30 minutes (Lightly)
		Friday	No workout			
		Saturday*	Workout			30 minutes (Lightly)
		Sunday	No workout			

A NEW HEALTHY YOU!
Workout Plan Schedule

DAY 21

Date	Week	Day	Exercise	Completed (x)	Weigh In	Workout Time
	1	Monday	No workout			
		Tuesday	Workout			30 minutes (Lightly)
		Wednesday	No workout			
		Thursday	Workout			30 minutes (Lightly)
		Friday	No workout			
		Saturday*	Workout			30 minutes (Lightly)
		Sunday	No workout			
	2	Monday	Workout			30 minutes (Lightly)
		Tuesday	No workout			
		Wednesday	Workout			30 minutes (Lightly)
		Thursday	No workout			
		Friday	Workout			30 minutes (Lightly)
		Saturday*	No workout			
		Sunday	Workout			30 minutes (Lightly)
	3	Monday	No workout			
		Tuesday	Workout			30 minutes (Lightly)
		Wednesday	No workout			
		Thursday	Workout			30 minutes (Lightly)
		Friday	No workout			
		Saturday*	Workout			30 minutes (Lightly)
		Sunday	No workout			

A NEW HEALTHY YOU!
Workout Plan Schedule

DAY 22

Date	Week	Day	Exercise	Completed (x)	Weigh In	Workout Time
	1	Monday	No workout			
		Tuesday	Workout			30 minutes (Lightly)
		Wednesday	No workout			
		Thursday	Workout			30 minutes (Lightly)
		Friday	No workout			
		Saturday*	Workout			30 minutes (Lightly)
		Sunday	No workout			
	2	Monday	Workout			30 minutes (Lightly)
		Tuesday	No workout			
		Wednesday	Workout			30 minutes (Lightly)
		Thursday	No workout			
		Friday	Workout			30 minutes (Lightly)
		Saturday*	No workout			
		Sunday	Workout			30 minutes (Lightly)
	3	Monday	No workout			
		Tuesday	Workout			30 minutes (Lightly)
		Wednesday	No workout			
		Thursday	Workout			30 minutes (Lightly)
		Friday	No workout			
		Saturday*	Workout			30 minutes (Lightly)
		Sunday	No workout			

A NEW HEALTHY YOU!
Workout Plan Schedule

DAY 23

Date	Week	Day	Exercise	Completed (x)	Weigh In	Workout Time
	1	Monday	No workout			
		Tuesday	Workout			30 minutes (Lightly)
		Wednesday	No workout			
		Thursday	Workout			30 minutes (Lightly)
		Friday	No workout			
		Saturday*	Workout			30 minutes (Lightly)
		Sunday	No workout			
	2	Monday	Workout			30 minutes (Lightly)
		Tuesday	No workout			
		Wednesday	Workout			30 minutes (Lightly)
		Thursday	No workout			
		Friday	Workout			30 minutes (Lightly)
		Saturday*	No workout			
		Sunday	Workout			30 minutes (Lightly)
	3	Monday	No workout			
		Tuesday	Workout			30 minutes (Lightly)
		Wednesday	No workout			
		Thursday	Workout			30 minutes (Lightly)
		Friday	No workout			
		Saturday*	Workout			30 minutes (Lightly)
		Sunday	No workout			

A NEW HEALTHY YOU!
Workout Plan Schedule

DAY 24

Date	Week	Day	Exercise	Completed (x)	Weigh In	Workout Time
	1	Monday	No workout			
		Tuesday	Workout			30 minutes (Lightly)
		Wednesday	No workout			
		Thursday	Workout			30 minutes (Lightly)
		Friday	No workout			
		Saturday*	Workout			30 minutes (Lightly)
		Sunday	No workout			
	2	Monday	Workout			30 minutes (Lightly)
		Tuesday	No workout			
		Wednesday	Workout			30 minutes (Lightly)
		Thursday	No workout			
		Friday	Workout			30 minutes (Lightly)
		Saturday*	No workout			
		Sunday	Workout			30 minutes (Lightly)
	3	Monday	No workout			
		Tuesday	Workout			30 minutes (Lightly)
		Wednesday	No workout			
		Thursday	Workout			30 minutes (Lightly)
		Friday	No workout			
		Saturday*	Workout			30 minutes (Lightly)
		Sunday	No workout			

A NEW HEALTHY YOU!
Workout Plan Schedule

DAY 25

Date	Week	Day	Exercise	Completed (x)	Weigh In	Workout Time
	1	Monday	No workout			
		Tuesday	Workout			30 minutes (Lightly)
		Wednesday	No workout			
		Thursday	Workout			30 minutes (Lightly)
		Friday	No workout			
		Saturday*	Workout			30 minutes (Lightly)
		Sunday	No workout			
	2	Monday	Workout			30 minutes (Lightly)
		Tuesday	No workout			
		Wednesday	Workout			30 minutes (Lightly)
		Thursday	No workout			
		Friday	Workout			30 minutes (Lightly)
		Saturday*	No workout			
		Sunday	Workout			30 minutes (Lightly)
	3	Monday	No workout			
		Tuesday	Workout			30 minutes (Lightly)
		Wednesday	No workout			
		Thursday	Workout			30 minutes (Lightly)
		Friday	No workout			
		Saturday*	Workout			30 minutes (Lightly)
		Sunday	No workout			

A NEW HEALTHY YOU!
Workout Plan Schedule

DAY 26

Date	Week	Day	Exercise	Completed (x)	Weigh In	Workout Time
	1	Monday	No workout			
		Tuesday	Workout			30 minutes (Lightly)
		Wednesday	No workout			
		Thursday	Workout			30 minutes (Lightly)
		Friday	No workout			
		Saturday*	Workout			30 minutes (Lightly)
		Sunday	No workout			
	2	Monday	Workout			30 minutes (Lightly)
		Tuesday	No workout			
		Wednesday	Workout			30 minutes (Lightly)
		Thursday	No workout			
		Friday	Workout			30 minutes (Lightly)
		Saturday*	No workout			
		Sunday	Workout			30 minutes (Lightly)
	3	Monday	No workout			
		Tuesday	Workout			30 minutes (Lightly)
		Wednesday	No workout			
		Thursday	Workout			30 minutes (Lightly)
		Friday	No workout			
		Saturday*	Workout			30 minutes (Lightly)
		Sunday	No workout			

A NEW HEALTHY YOU!
Workout Plan Schedule

DAY 27

Date	Week	Day	Exercise	Completed (x)	Weigh In	Workout Time
	1	Monday	No workout			
		Tuesday	Workout			30 minutes (Lightly)
		Wednesday	No workout			
		Thursday	Workout			30 minutes (Lightly)
		Friday	No workout			
		Saturday*	Workout			30 minutes (Lightly)
		Sunday	No workout			
	2	Monday	Workout			30 minutes (Lightly)
		Tuesday	No workout			
		Wednesday	Workout			30 minutes (Lightly)
		Thursday	No workout			
		Friday	Workout			30 minutes (Lightly)
		Saturday*	No workout			
		Sunday	Workout			30 minutes (Lightly)
	3	Monday	No workout			
		Tuesday	Workout			30 minutes (Lightly)
		Wednesday	No workout			
		Thursday	Workout			30 minutes (Lightly)
		Friday	No workout			
		Saturday*	Workout			30 minutes (Lightly)
		Sunday	No workout			

A NEW HEALTHY YOU!
Workout Plan Schedule

DAY 28

Date	Week	Day	Exercise	Completed (x)	Weigh In	Workout Time
	1	Monday	No workout			
		Tuesday	Workout			30 minutes (Lightly)
		Wednesday	No workout			
		Thursday	Workout			30 minutes (Lightly)
		Friday	No workout			
		Saturday*	Workout			30 minutes (Lightly)
		Sunday	No workout			
	2	Monday	Workout			30 minutes (Lightly)
		Tuesday	No workout			
		Wednesday	Workout			30 minutes (Lightly)
		Thursday	No workout			
		Friday	Workout			30 minutes (Lightly)
		Saturday*	No workout			
		Sunday	Workout			30 minutes (Lightly)
	3	Monday	No workout			
		Tuesday	Workout			30 minutes (Lightly)
		Wednesday	No workout			
		Thursday	Workout			30 minutes (Lightly)
		Friday	No workout			
		Saturday*	Workout			30 minutes (Lightly)
		Sunday	No workout			

A NEW HEALTHY YOU!
Workout Plan Schedule

DAY 29

Date	Week	Day	Exercise	Completed (x)	Weigh In	Workout Time
	1	Monday	No workout			
		Tuesday	Workout			30 minutes (Lightly)
		Wednesday	No workout			
		Thursday	Workout			30 minutes (Lightly)
		Friday	No workout			
		Saturday*	Workout			30 minutes (Lightly)
		Sunday	No workout			
	2	Monday	Workout			30 minutes (Lightly)
		Tuesday	No workout			
		Wednesday	Workout			30 minutes (Lightly)
		Thursday	No workout			
		Friday	Workout			30 minutes (Lightly)
		Saturday*	No workout			
		Sunday	Workout			30 minutes (Lightly)
	3	Monday	No workout			
		Tuesday	Workout			30 minutes (Lightly)
		Wednesday	No workout			
		Thursday	Workout			30 minutes (Lightly)
		Friday	No workout			
		Saturday*	Workout			30 minutes (Lightly)
		Sunday	No workout			

A NEW HEALTHY YOU!
Workout Plan Schedule

DAY 30

Date	Week	Day	Exercise	Completed (x)	Weigh In	Workout Time
	1	Monday	No workout			
		Tuesday	Workout			30 minutes (Lightly)
		Wednesday	No workout			
		Thursday	Workout			30 minutes (Lightly)
		Friday	No workout			
		Saturday*	Workout			30 minutes (Lightly)
		Sunday	No workout			
	2	Monday	Workout			30 minutes (Lightly)
		Tuesday	No workout			
		Wednesday	Workout			30 minutes (Lightly)
		Thursday	No workout			
		Friday	Workout			30 minutes (Lightly)
		Saturday*	No workout			
		Sunday	Workout			30 minutes (Lightly)
	3	Monday	No workout			
		Tuesday	Workout			30 minutes (Lightly)
		Wednesday	No workout			
		Thursday	Workout			30 minutes (Lightly)
		Friday	No workout			
		Saturday*	Workout			30 minutes (Lightly)
		Sunday	No workout			

A NEW HEALTHY YOU!
Workout Plan Schedule

DAY 31

Date	Week	Day	Exercise	Completed (x)	Weigh In	Workout Time
	1	Monday	No workout			
		Tuesday	Workout			30 minutes (Lightly)
		Wednesday	No workout			
		Thursday	Workout			30 minutes (Lightly)
		Friday	No workout			
		Saturday*	Workout			30 minutes (Lightly)
		Sunday	No workout			
	2	Monday	Workout			30 minutes (Lightly)
		Tuesday	No workout			
		Wednesday	Workout			30 minutes (Lightly)
		Thursday	No workout			
		Friday	Workout			30 minutes (Lightly)
		Saturday*	No workout			
		Sunday	Workout			30 minutes (Lightly)
	3	Monday	No workout			
		Tuesday	Workout			30 minutes (Lightly)
		Wednesday	No workout			
		Thursday	Workout			30 minutes (Lightly)
		Friday	No workout			
		Saturday*	Workout			30 minutes (Lightly)
		Sunday	No workout			

A NEW HEALTHY YOU!
Workout Plan Schedule

DAY 32

Date	Week	Day	Exercise	Completed (x)	Weigh In	Workout Time
	1	Monday	No workout			
		Tuesday	Workout			30 minutes (Lightly)
		Wednesday	No workout			
		Thursday	Workout			30 minutes (Lightly)
		Friday	No workout			
		Saturday*	Workout			30 minutes (Lightly)
		Sunday	No workout			
	2	Monday	Workout			30 minutes (Lightly)
		Tuesday	No workout			
		Wednesday	Workout			30 minutes (Lightly)
		Thursday	No workout			
		Friday	Workout			30 minutes (Lightly)
		Saturday*	No workout			
		Sunday	Workout			30 minutes (Lightly)
	3	Monday	No workout			
		Tuesday	Workout			30 minutes (Lightly)
		Wednesday	No workout			
		Thursday	Workout			30 minutes (Lightly)
		Friday	No workout			
		Saturday*	Workout			30 minutes (Lightly)
		Sunday	No workout			

A NEW HEALTHY YOU!
Workout Plan Schedule

DAY 33

Date	Week	Day	Exercise	Completed (x)	Weigh In	Workout Time
	1	Monday	No workout			
		Tuesday	Workout			30 minutes (Lightly)
		Wednesday	No workout			
		Thursday	Workout			30 minutes (Lightly)
		Friday	No workout			
		Saturday*	Workout			30 minutes (Lightly)
		Sunday	No workout			
	2	Monday	Workout			30 minutes (Lightly)
		Tuesday	No workout			
		Wednesday	Workout			30 minutes (Lightly)
		Thursday	No workout			
		Friday	Workout			30 minutes (Lightly)
		Saturday*	No workout			
		Sunday	Workout			30 minutes (Lightly)
	3	Monday	No workout			
		Tuesday	Workout			30 minutes (Lightly)
		Wednesday	No workout			
		Thursday	Workout			30 minutes (Lightly)
		Friday	No workout			
		Saturday*	Workout			30 minutes (Lightly)
		Sunday	No workout			

A NEW HEALTHY YOU!
Workout Plan Schedule

DAY 34

Date	Week	Day	Exercise	Completed (x)	Weigh In	Workout Time
	1	Monday	No workout			
		Tuesday	Workout			30 minutes (Lightly)
		Wednesday	No workout			
		Thursday	Workout			30 minutes (Lightly)
		Friday	No workout			
		Saturday*	Workout			30 minutes (Lightly)
		Sunday	No workout			
	2	Monday	Workout			30 minutes (Lightly)
		Tuesday	No workout			
		Wednesday	Workout			30 minutes (Lightly)
		Thursday	No workout			
		Friday	Workout			30 minutes (Lightly)
		Saturday*	No workout			
		Sunday	Workout			30 minutes (Lightly)
	3	Monday	No workout			
		Tuesday	Workout			30 minutes (Lightly)
		Wednesday	No workout			
		Thursday	Workout			30 minutes (Lightly)
		Friday	No workout			
		Saturday*	Workout			30 minutes (Lightly)
		Sunday	No workout			

A NEW HEALTHY YOU!
Workout Plan Schedule

DAY 35

Date	Week	Day	Exercise	Completed (x)	Weigh In	Workout Time
	1	Monday	No workout			
		Tuesday	Workout			30 minutes (Lightly)
		Wednesday	No workout			
		Thursday	Workout			30 minutes (Lightly)
		Friday	No workout			
		Saturday*	Workout			30 minutes (Lightly)
		Sunday	No workout			
	2	Monday	Workout			30 minutes (Lightly)
		Tuesday	No workout			
		Wednesday	Workout			30 minutes (Lightly)
		Thursday	No workout			
		Friday	Workout			30 minutes (Lightly)
		Saturday*	No workout			
		Sunday	Workout			30 minutes (Lightly)
	3	Monday	No workout			
		Tuesday	Workout			30 minutes (Lightly)
		Wednesday	No workout			
		Thursday	Workout			30 minutes (Lightly)
		Friday	No workout			
		Saturday*	Workout			30 minutes (Lightly)
		Sunday	No workout			

A NEW HEALTHY YOU!
Workout Plan Schedule

DAY 36

Date	Week	Day	Exercise	Completed (x)	Weigh In	Workout Time
	1	Monday	No workout			
		Tuesday	Workout			30 minutes (Lightly)
		Wednesday	No workout			
		Thursday	Workout			30 minutes (Lightly)
		Friday	No workout			
		Saturday*	Workout			30 minutes (Lightly)
		Sunday	No workout			
	2	Monday	Workout			30 minutes (Lightly)
		Tuesday	No workout			
		Wednesday	Workout			30 minutes (Lightly)
		Thursday	No workout			
		Friday	Workout			30 minutes (Lightly)
		Saturday*	No workout			
		Sunday	Workout			30 minutes (Lightly)
	3	Monday	No workout			
		Tuesday	Workout			30 minutes (Lightly)
		Wednesday	No workout			
		Thursday	Workout			30 minutes (Lightly)
		Friday	No workout			
		Saturday*	Workout			30 minutes (Lightly)
		Sunday	No workout			

A NEW HEALTHY YOU!
Workout Plan Schedule

DAY 37

Date	Week	Day	Exercise	Completed (x)	Weigh In	Workout Time
	1	Monday	No workout			
		Tuesday	Workout			30 minutes (Lightly)
		Wednesday	No workout			
		Thursday	Workout			30 minutes (Lightly)
		Friday	No workout			
		Saturday*	Workout			30 minutes (Lightly)
		Sunday	No workout			
	2	Monday	Workout			30 minutes (Lightly)
		Tuesday	No workout			
		Wednesday	Workout			30 minutes (Lightly)
		Thursday	No workout			
		Friday	Workout			30 minutes (Lightly)
		Saturday*	No workout			
		Sunday	Workout			30 minutes (Lightly)
	3	Monday	No workout			
		Tuesday	Workout			30 minutes (Lightly)
		Wednesday	No workout			
		Thursday	Workout			30 minutes (Lightly)
		Friday	No workout			
		Saturday*	Workout			30 minutes (Lightly)
		Sunday	No workout			

A NEW HEALTHY YOU!
Workout Plan Schedule

DAY 38

Date	Week	Day	Exercise	Completed (x)	Weigh In	Workout Time
	1	Monday	No workout			
		Tuesday	Workout			30 minutes (Lightly)
		Wednesday	No workout			
		Thursday	Workout			30 minutes (Lightly)
		Friday	No workout			
		Saturday*	Workout			30 minutes (Lightly)
		Sunday	No workout			
	2	Monday	Workout			30 minutes (Lightly)
		Tuesday	No workout			
		Wednesday	Workout			30 minutes (Lightly)
		Thursday	No workout			
		Friday	Workout			30 minutes (Lightly)
		Saturday*	No workout			
		Sunday	Workout			30 minutes (Lightly)
	3	Monday	No workout			
		Tuesday	Workout			30 minutes (Lightly)
		Wednesday	No workout			
		Thursday	Workout			30 minutes (Lightly)
		Friday	No workout			
		Saturday*	Workout			30 minutes (Lightly)
		Sunday	No workout			

A NEW HEALTHY YOU!
Workout Plan Schedule

DAY 39

Date	Week	Day	Exercise	Completed (x)	Weigh In	Workout Time
	1	Monday	No workout			
		Tuesday	Workout			30 minutes (Lightly)
		Wednesday	No workout			
		Thursday	Workout			30 minutes (Lightly)
		Friday	No workout			
		Saturday*	Workout			30 minutes (Lightly)
		Sunday	No workout			
	2	Monday	Workout			30 minutes (Lightly)
		Tuesday	No workout			
		Wednesday	Workout			30 minutes (Lightly)
		Thursday	No workout			
		Friday	Workout			30 minutes (Lightly)
		Saturday*	No workout			
		Sunday	Workout			30 minutes (Lightly)
	3	Monday	No workout			
		Tuesday	Workout			30 minutes (Lightly)
		Wednesday	No workout			
		Thursday	Workout			30 minutes (Lightly)
		Friday	No workout			
		Saturday*	Workout			30 minutes (Lightly)
		Sunday	No workout			

A NEW HEALTHY YOU!
Workout Plan Schedule

DAY 40

Date	Week	Day	Exercise	Completed (x)	Weigh In	Workout Time
	1	Monday	No workout			
		Tuesday	Workout			30 minutes (Lightly)
		Wednesday	No workout			
		Thursday	Workout			30 minutes (Lightly)
		Friday	No workout			
		Saturday*	Workout			30 minutes (Lightly)
		Sunday	No workout			
	2	Monday	Workout			30 minutes (Lightly)
		Tuesday	No workout			
		Wednesday	Workout			30 minutes (Lightly)
		Thursday	No workout			
		Friday	Workout			30 minutes (Lightly)
		Saturday*	No workout			
		Sunday	Workout			30 minutes (Lightly)
	3	Monday	No workout			
		Tuesday	Workout			30 minutes (Lightly)
		Wednesday	No workout			
		Thursday	Workout			30 minutes (Lightly)
		Friday	No workout			
		Saturday*	Workout			30 minutes (Lightly)
		Sunday	No workout			

A NEW HEALTHY YOU!
Workout Plan Schedule

DAY 41

Date	Week	Day	Exercise	Completed (x)	Weigh In	Workout Time
	1	Monday	No workout			
		Tuesday	Workout			30 minutes (Lightly)
		Wednesday	No workout			
		Thursday	Workout			30 minutes (Lightly)
		Friday	No workout			
		Saturday*	Workout			30 minutes (Lightly)
		Sunday	No workout			
	2	Monday	Workout			30 minutes (Lightly)
		Tuesday	No workout			
		Wednesday	Workout			30 minutes (Lightly)
		Thursday	No workout			
		Friday	Workout			30 minutes (Lightly)
		Saturday*	No workout			
		Sunday	Workout			30 minutes (Lightly)
	3	Monday	No workout			
		Tuesday	Workout			30 minutes (Lightly)
		Wednesday	No workout			
		Thursday	Workout			30 minutes (Lightly)
		Friday	No workout			
		Saturday*	Workout			30 minutes (Lightly)
		Sunday	No workout			

A NEW HEALTHY YOU!
Workout Plan Schedule

DAY 42

Date	Week	Day	Exercise	Completed (x)	Weigh In	Workout Time
	1	Monday	No workout			
		Tuesday	Workout			30 minutes (Lightly)
		Wednesday	No workout			
		Thursday	Workout			30 minutes (Lightly)
		Friday	No workout			
		Saturday*	Workout			30 minutes (Lightly)
		Sunday	No workout			
	2	Monday	Workout			30 minutes (Lightly)
		Tuesday	No workout			
		Wednesday	Workout			30 minutes (Lightly)
		Thursday	No workout			
		Friday	Workout			30 minutes (Lightly)
		Saturday*	No workout			
		Sunday	Workout			30 minutes (Lightly)
	3	Monday	No workout			
		Tuesday	Workout			30 minutes (Lightly)
		Wednesday	No workout			
		Thursday	Workout			30 minutes (Lightly)
		Friday	No workout			
		Saturday*	Workout			30 minutes (Lightly)
		Sunday	No workout			

A NEW HEALTHY YOU!
Workout Plan Schedule

DAY 43

Date	Week	Day	Exercise	Completed (x)	Weigh In	Workout Time
	1	Monday	No workout			
		Tuesday	Workout			30 minutes (Lightly)
		Wednesday	No workout			
		Thursday	Workout			30 minutes (Lightly)
		Friday	No workout			
		Saturday*	Workout			30 minutes (Lightly)
		Sunday	No workout			
	2	Monday	Workout			30 minutes (Lightly)
		Tuesday	No workout			
		Wednesday	Workout			30 minutes (Lightly)
		Thursday	No workout			
		Friday	Workout			30 minutes (Lightly)
		Saturday*	No workout			
		Sunday	Workout			30 minutes (Lightly)
	3	Monday	No workout			
		Tuesday	Workout			30 minutes (Lightly)
		Wednesday	No workout			
		Thursday	Workout			30 minutes (Lightly)
		Friday	No workout			
		Saturday*	Workout			30 minutes (Lightly)
		Sunday	No workout			

A NEW HEALTHY YOU!
Workout Plan Schedule

DAY 44

Date	Week	Day	Exercise	Completed (x)	Weigh In	Workout Time
	1	Monday	No workout			
		Tuesday	Workout			30 minutes (Lightly)
		Wednesday	No workout			
		Thursday	Workout			30 minutes (Lightly)
		Friday	No workout			
		Saturday*	Workout			30 minutes (Lightly)
		Sunday	No workout			
	2	Monday	Workout			30 minutes (Lightly)
		Tuesday	No workout			
		Wednesday	Workout			30 minutes (Lightly)
		Thursday	No workout			
		Friday	Workout			30 minutes (Lightly)
		Saturday*	No workout			
		Sunday	Workout			30 minutes (Lightly)
	3	Monday	No workout			
		Tuesday	Workout			30 minutes (Lightly)
		Wednesday	No workout			
		Thursday	Workout			30 minutes (Lightly)
		Friday	No workout			
		Saturday*	Workout			30 minutes (Lightly)
		Sunday	No workout			

A NEW HEALTHY YOU!
Workout Plan Schedule

DAY 45

Date	Week	Day	Exercise	Completed (x)	Weigh In	Workout Time
	1	Monday	No workout			
		Tuesday	Workout			30 minutes (Lightly)
		Wednesday	No workout			
		Thursday	Workout			30 minutes (Lightly)
		Friday	No workout			
		Saturday*	Workout			30 minutes (Lightly)
		Sunday	No workout			
	2	Monday	Workout			30 minutes (Lightly)
		Tuesday	No workout			
		Wednesday	Workout			30 minutes (Lightly)
		Thursday	No workout			
		Friday	Workout			30 minutes (Lightly)
		Saturday*	No workout			
		Sunday	Workout			30 minutes (Lightly)
	3	Monday	No workout			
		Tuesday	Workout			30 minutes (Lightly)
		Wednesday	No workout			
		Thursday	Workout			30 minutes (Lightly)
		Friday	No workout			
		Saturday*	Workout			30 minutes (Lightly)
		Sunday	No workout			

A NEW HEALTHY YOU!
Workout Plan Schedule

DAY 46

Date	Week	Day	Exercise	Completed (x)	Weigh In	Workout Time
	1	Monday	No workout			
		Tuesday	Workout			30 minutes (Lightly)
		Wednesday	No workout			
		Thursday	Workout			30 minutes (Lightly)
		Friday	No workout			
		Saturday*	Workout			30 minutes (Lightly)
		Sunday	No workout			
	2	Monday	Workout			30 minutes (Lightly)
		Tuesday	No workout			
		Wednesday	Workout			30 minutes (Lightly)
		Thursday	No workout			
		Friday	Workout			30 minutes (Lightly)
		Saturday*	No workout			
		Sunday	Workout			30 minutes (Lightly)
	3	Monday	No workout			
		Tuesday	Workout			30 minutes (Lightly)
		Wednesday	No workout			
		Thursday	Workout			30 minutes (Lightly)
		Friday	No workout			
		Saturday*	Workout			30 minutes (Lightly)
		Sunday	No workout			

A NEW HEALTHY YOU!
Workout Plan Schedule

DAY 47

Date	Week	Day	Exercise	Completed (x)	Weigh In	Workout Time
	1	Monday	No workout			
		Tuesday	Workout			30 minutes (Lightly)
		Wednesday	No workout			
		Thursday	Workout			30 minutes (Lightly)
		Friday	No workout			
		Saturday*	Workout			30 minutes (Lightly)
		Sunday	No workout			
	2	Monday	Workout			30 minutes (Lightly)
		Tuesday	No workout			
		Wednesday	Workout			30 minutes (Lightly)
		Thursday	No workout			
		Friday	Workout			30 minutes (Lightly)
		Saturday*	No workout			
		Sunday	Workout			30 minutes (Lightly)
	3	Monday	No workout			
		Tuesday	Workout			30 minutes (Lightly)
		Wednesday	No workout			
		Thursday	Workout			30 minutes (Lightly)
		Friday	No workout			
		Saturday*	Workout			30 minutes (Lightly)
		Sunday	No workout			

A NEW HEALTHY YOU!
Workout Plan Schedule

DAY 48

Date	Week	Day	Exercise	Completed (x)	Weigh In	Workout Time
	1	Monday	No workout			
		Tuesday	Workout			30 minutes (Lightly)
		Wednesday	No workout			
		Thursday	Workout			30 minutes (Lightly)
		Friday	No workout			
		Saturday*	Workout			30 minutes (Lightly)
		Sunday	No workout			
	2	Monday	Workout			30 minutes (Lightly)
		Tuesday	No workout			
		Wednesday	Workout			30 minutes (Lightly)
		Thursday	No workout			
		Friday	Workout			30 minutes (Lightly)
		Saturday*	No workout			
		Sunday	Workout			30 minutes (Lightly)
	3	Monday	No workout			
		Tuesday	Workout			30 minutes (Lightly)
		Wednesday	No workout			
		Thursday	Workout			30 minutes (Lightly)
		Friday	No workout			
		Saturday*	Workout			30 minutes (Lightly)
		Sunday	No workout			

A NEW HEALTHY YOU!
Workout Plan Schedule

DAY 49

Date	Week	Day	Exercise	Completed (x)	Weigh In	Workout Time
	1	Monday	No workout			
		Tuesday	Workout			30 minutes (Lightly)
		Wednesday	No workout			
		Thursday	Workout			30 minutes (Lightly)
		Friday	No workout			
		Saturday*	Workout			30 minutes (Lightly)
		Sunday	No workout			
	2	Monday	Workout			30 minutes (Lightly)
		Tuesday	No workout			
		Wednesday	Workout			30 minutes (Lightly)
		Thursday	No workout			
		Friday	Workout			30 minutes (Lightly)
		Saturday*	No workout			
		Sunday	Workout			30 minutes (Lightly)
	3	Monday	No workout			
		Tuesday	Workout			30 minutes (Lightly)
		Wednesday	No workout			
		Thursday	Workout			30 minutes (Lightly)
		Friday	No workout			
		Saturday*	Workout			30 minutes (Lightly)
		Sunday	No workout			

A NEW HEALTHY YOU!
Workout Plan Schedule

DAY 50

Date	Week	Day	Exercise	Completed (x)	Weigh In	Workout Time
	1	Monday	No workout			
		Tuesday	Workout			30 minutes (Lightly)
		Wednesday	No workout			
		Thursday	Workout			30 minutes (Lightly)
		Friday	No workout			
		Saturday*	Workout			30 minutes (Lightly)
		Sunday	No workout			
	2	Monday	Workout			30 minutes (Lightly)
		Tuesday	No workout			
		Wednesday	Workout			30 minutes (Lightly)
		Thursday	No workout			
		Friday	Workout			30 minutes (Lightly)
		Saturday*	No workout			
		Sunday	Workout			30 minutes (Lightly)
	3	Monday	No workout			
		Tuesday	Workout			30 minutes (Lightly)
		Wednesday	No workout			
		Thursday	Workout			30 minutes (Lightly)
		Friday	No workout			
		Saturday*	Workout			30 minutes (Lightly)
		Sunday	No workout			

A NEW HEALTHY YOU!
Workout Plan Schedule

DAY 51

Date	Week	Day	Exercise	Completed (x)	Weigh In	Workout Time
	1	Monday	No workout			
		Tuesday	Workout			30 minutes (Lightly)
		Wednesday	No workout			
		Thursday	Workout			30 minutes (Lightly)
		Friday	No workout			
		Saturday*	Workout			30 minutes (Lightly)
		Sunday	No workout			
	2	Monday	Workout			30 minutes (Lightly)
		Tuesday	No workout			
		Wednesday	Workout			30 minutes (Lightly)
		Thursday	No workout			
		Friday	Workout			30 minutes (Lightly)
		Saturday*	No workout			
		Sunday	Workout			30 minutes (Lightly)
	3	Monday	No workout			
		Tuesday	Workout			30 minutes (Lightly)
		Wednesday	No workout			
		Thursday	Workout			30 minutes (Lightly)
		Friday	No workout			
		Saturday*	Workout			30 minutes (Lightly)
		Sunday	No workout			

A NEW HEALTHY YOU!
Workout Plan Schedule

DAY 52

Date	Week	Day	Exercise	Completed (x)	Weigh In	Workout Time
	1	Monday	No workout			
		Tuesday	Workout			30 minutes (Lightly)
		Wednesday	No workout			
		Thursday	Workout			30 minutes (Lightly)
		Friday	No workout			
		Saturday*	Workout			30 minutes (Lightly)
		Sunday	No workout			
	2	Monday	Workout			30 minutes (Lightly)
		Tuesday	No workout			
		Wednesday	Workout			30 minutes (Lightly)
		Thursday	No workout			
		Friday	Workout			30 minutes (Lightly)
		Saturday*	No workout			
		Sunday	Workout			30 minutes (Lightly)
	3	Monday	No workout			
		Tuesday	Workout			30 minutes (Lightly)
		Wednesday	No workout			
		Thursday	Workout			30 minutes (Lightly)
		Friday	No workout			
		Saturday*	Workout			30 minutes (Lightly)
		Sunday	No workout			

A NEW HEALTHY YOU!
Workout Plan Schedule

DAY 53

Date	Week	Day	Exercise	Completed (x)	Weigh In	Workout Time
	1	Monday	No workout			
		Tuesday	Workout			30 minutes (Lightly)
		Wednesday	No workout			
		Thursday	Workout			30 minutes (Lightly)
		Friday	No workout			
		Saturday*	Workout			30 minutes (Lightly)
		Sunday	No workout			
	2	Monday	Workout			30 minutes (Lightly)
		Tuesday	No workout			
		Wednesday	Workout			30 minutes (Lightly)
		Thursday	No workout			
		Friday	Workout			30 minutes (Lightly)
		Saturday*	No workout			
		Sunday	Workout			30 minutes (Lightly)
	3	Monday	No workout			
		Tuesday	Workout			30 minutes (Lightly)
		Wednesday	No workout			
		Thursday	Workout			30 minutes (Lightly)
		Friday	No workout			
		Saturday*	Workout			30 minutes (Lightly)
		Sunday	No workout			

A NEW HEALTHY YOU!
Workout Plan Schedule

DAY 54

Date	Week	Day	Exercise	Completed (x)	Weigh In	Workout Time
	1	Monday	No workout			
		Tuesday	Workout			30 minutes (Lightly)
		Wednesday	No workout			
		Thursday	Workout			30 minutes (Lightly)
		Friday	No workout			
		Saturday*	Workout			30 minutes (Lightly)
		Sunday	No workout			
	2	Monday	Workout			30 minutes (Lightly)
		Tuesday	No workout			
		Wednesday	Workout			30 minutes (Lightly)
		Thursday	No workout			
		Friday	Workout			30 minutes (Lightly)
		Saturday*	No workout			
		Sunday	Workout			30 minutes (Lightly)
	3	Monday	No workout			
		Tuesday	Workout			30 minutes (Lightly)
		Wednesday	No workout			
		Thursday	Workout			30 minutes (Lightly)
		Friday	No workout			
		Saturday*	Workout			30 minutes (Lightly)
		Sunday	No workout			

A NEW HEALTHY YOU!
Workout Plan Schedule

DAY 55

Date	Week	Day	Exercise	Completed (x)	Weigh In	Workout Time
	1	Monday	No workout			
		Tuesday	Workout			30 minutes (Lightly)
		Wednesday	No workout			
		Thursday	Workout			30 minutes (Lightly)
		Friday	No workout			
		Saturday*	Workout			30 minutes (Lightly)
		Sunday	No workout			
	2	Monday	Workout			30 minutes (Lightly)
		Tuesday	No workout			
		Wednesday	Workout			30 minutes (Lightly)
		Thursday	No workout			
		Friday	Workout			30 minutes (Lightly)
		Saturday*	No workout			
		Sunday	Workout			30 minutes (Lightly)
	3	Monday	No workout			
		Tuesday	Workout			30 minutes (Lightly)
		Wednesday	No workout			
		Thursday	Workout			30 minutes (Lightly)
		Friday	No workout			
		Saturday*	Workout			30 minutes (Lightly)
		Sunday	No workout			

A NEW HEALTHY YOU!
Workout Plan Schedule

DAY 56

Date	Week	Day	Exercise	Completed (x)	Weigh In	Workout Time
	1	Monday	No workout			
		Tuesday	Workout			30 minutes (Lightly)
		Wednesday	No workout			
		Thursday	Workout			30 minutes (Lightly)
		Friday	No workout			
		Saturday*	Workout			30 minutes (Lightly)
		Sunday	No workout			
	2	Monday	Workout			30 minutes (Lightly)
		Tuesday	No workout			
		Wednesday	Workout			30 minutes (Lightly)
		Thursday	No workout			
		Friday	Workout			30 minutes (Lightly)
		Saturday*	No workout			
		Sunday	Workout			30 minutes (Lightly)
	3	Monday	No workout			
		Tuesday	Workout			30 minutes (Lightly)
		Wednesday	No workout			
		Thursday	Workout			30 minutes (Lightly)
		Friday	No workout			
		Saturday*	Workout			30 minutes (Lightly)
		Sunday	No workout			

A NEW HEALTHY YOU!
Workout Plan Schedule

DAY 57

Date	Week	Day	Exercise	Completed (x)	Weigh In	Workout Time
	1	Monday	No workout			
		Tuesday	Workout			30 minutes (Lightly)
		Wednesday	No workout			
		Thursday	Workout			30 minutes (Lightly)
		Friday	No workout			
		Saturday*	Workout			30 minutes (Lightly)
		Sunday	No workout			
	2	Monday	Workout			30 minutes (Lightly)
		Tuesday	No workout			
		Wednesday	Workout			30 minutes (Lightly)
		Thursday	No workout			
		Friday	Workout			30 minutes (Lightly)
		Saturday*	No workout			
		Sunday	Workout			30 minutes (Lightly)
	3	Monday	No workout			
		Tuesday	Workout			30 minutes (Lightly)
		Wednesday	No workout			
		Thursday	Workout			30 minutes (Lightly)
		Friday	No workout			
		Saturday*	Workout			30 minutes (Lightly)
		Sunday	No workout			

A NEW HEALTHY YOU!
Workout Plan Schedule

DAY 58

Date	Week	Day	Exercise	Completed (x)	Weigh In	Workout Time
	1	Monday	No workout			
		Tuesday	Workout			30 minutes (Lightly)
		Wednesday	No workout			
		Thursday	Workout			30 minutes (Lightly)
		Friday	No workout			
		Saturday*	Workout			30 minutes (Lightly)
		Sunday	No workout			
	2	Monday	Workout			30 minutes (Lightly)
		Tuesday	No workout			
		Wednesday	Workout			30 minutes (Lightly)
		Thursday	No workout			
		Friday	Workout			30 minutes (Lightly)
		Saturday*	No workout			
		Sunday	Workout			30 minutes (Lightly)
	3	Monday	No workout			
		Tuesday	Workout			30 minutes (Lightly)
		Wednesday	No workout			
		Thursday	Workout			30 minutes (Lightly)
		Friday	No workout			
		Saturday*	Workout			30 minutes (Lightly)
		Sunday	No workout			

A NEW HEALTHY YOU!
Workout Plan Schedule

DAY 59

Date	Week	Day	Exercise	Completed (x)	Weigh In	Workout Time
	1	Monday	No workout			
		Tuesday	Workout			30 minutes (Lightly)
		Wednesday	No workout			
		Thursday	Workout			30 minutes (Lightly)
		Friday	No workout			
		Saturday*	Workout			30 minutes (Lightly)
		Sunday	No workout			
	2	Monday	Workout			30 minutes (Lightly)
		Tuesday	No workout			
		Wednesday	Workout			30 minutes (Lightly)
		Thursday	No workout			
		Friday	Workout			30 minutes (Lightly)
		Saturday*	No workout			
		Sunday	Workout			30 minutes (Lightly)
	3	Monday	No workout			
		Tuesday	Workout			30 minutes (Lightly)
		Wednesday	No workout			
		Thursday	Workout			30 minutes (Lightly)
		Friday	No workout			
		Saturday*	Workout			30 minutes (Lightly)
		Sunday	No workout			

A NEW HEALTHY YOU!
Workout Plan Schedule

DAY 60

Date	Week	Day	Exercise	Completed (x)	Weigh In	Workout Time
	1	Monday	No workout			
		Tuesday	Workout			30 minutes (Lightly)
		Wednesday	No workout			
		Thursday	Workout			30 minutes (Lightly)
		Friday	No workout			
		Saturday*	Workout			30 minutes (Lightly)
		Sunday	No workout			
	2	Monday	Workout			30 minutes (Lightly)
		Tuesday	No workout			
		Wednesday	Workout			30 minutes (Lightly)
		Thursday	No workout			
		Friday	Workout			30 minutes (Lightly)
		Saturday*	No workout			
		Sunday	Workout			30 minutes (Lightly)
	3	Monday	No workout			
		Tuesday	Workout			30 minutes (Lightly)
		Wednesday	No workout			
		Thursday	Workout			30 minutes (Lightly)
		Friday	No workout			
		Saturday*	Workout			30 minutes (Lightly)
		Sunday	No workout			

A NEW HEALTHY YOU!
Workout Plan Schedule

DAY 61

Date	Week	Day	Exercise	Completed (x)	Weigh In	Workout Time
	1	Monday	No workout			
		Tuesday	Workout			30 minutes (Lightly)
		Wednesday	No workout			
		Thursday	Workout			30 minutes (Lightly)
		Friday	No workout			
		Saturday*	Workout			30 minutes (Lightly)
		Sunday	No workout			
	2	Monday	Workout			30 minutes (Lightly)
		Tuesday	No workout			
		Wednesday	Workout			30 minutes (Lightly)
		Thursday	No workout			
		Friday	Workout			30 minutes (Lightly)
		Saturday*	No workout			
		Sunday	Workout			30 minutes (Lightly)
	3	Monday	No workout			
		Tuesday	Workout			30 minutes (Lightly)
		Wednesday	No workout			
		Thursday	Workout			30 minutes (Lightly)
		Friday	No workout			
		Saturday*	Workout			30 minutes (Lightly)
		Sunday	No workout			

A NEW HEALTHY YOU!
Workout Plan Schedule

DAY 62

Date	Week	Day	Exercise	Completed (x)	Weigh In	Workout Time
	1	Monday	No workout			
		Tuesday	Workout			30 minutes (Lightly)
		Wednesday	No workout			
		Thursday	Workout			30 minutes (Lightly)
		Friday	No workout			
		Saturday*	Workout			30 minutes (Lightly)
		Sunday	No workout			
	2	Monday	Workout			30 minutes (Lightly)
		Tuesday	No workout			
		Wednesday	Workout			30 minutes (Lightly)
		Thursday	No workout			
		Friday	Workout			30 minutes (Lightly)
		Saturday*	No workout			
		Sunday	Workout			30 minutes (Lightly)
	3	Monday	No workout			
		Tuesday	Workout			30 minutes (Lightly)
		Wednesday	No workout			
		Thursday	Workout			30 minutes (Lightly)
		Friday	No workout			
		Saturday*	Workout			30 minutes (Lightly)
		Sunday	No workout			

A NEW HEALTHY YOU!
Workout Plan Schedule

DAY 63

Date	Week	Day	Exercise	Completed (x)	Weigh In	Workout Time
	1	Monday	No workout			
		Tuesday	Workout			30 minutes (Lightly)
		Wednesday	No workout			
		Thursday	Workout			30 minutes (Lightly)
		Friday	No workout			
		Saturday*	Workout			30 minutes (Lightly)
		Sunday	No workout			
	2	Monday	Workout			30 minutes (Lightly)
		Tuesday	No workout			
		Wednesday	Workout			30 minutes (Lightly)
		Thursday	No workout			
		Friday	Workout			30 minutes (Lightly)
		Saturday*	No workout			
		Sunday	Workout			30 minutes (Lightly)
	3	Monday	No workout			
		Tuesday	Workout			30 minutes (Lightly)
		Wednesday	No workout			
		Thursday	Workout			30 minutes (Lightly)
		Friday	No workout			
		Saturday*	Workout			30 minutes (Lightly)
		Sunday	No workout			

A NEW HEALTHY YOU!
Workout Plan Schedule

DAY 64

Date	Week	Day	Exercise	Completed (x)	Weigh In	Workout Time
	1	Monday	No workout			
		Tuesday	Workout			30 minutes (Lightly)
		Wednesday	No workout			
		Thursday	Workout			30 minutes (Lightly)
		Friday	No workout			
		Saturday*	Workout			30 minutes (Lightly)
		Sunday	No workout			
	2	Monday	Workout			30 minutes (Lightly)
		Tuesday	No workout			
		Wednesday	Workout			30 minutes (Lightly)
		Thursday	No workout			
		Friday	Workout			30 minutes (Lightly)
		Saturday*	No workout			
		Sunday	Workout			30 minutes (Lightly)
	3	Monday	No workout			
		Tuesday	Workout			30 minutes (Lightly)
		Wednesday	No workout			
		Thursday	Workout			30 minutes (Lightly)
		Friday	No workout			
		Saturday*	Workout			30 minutes (Lightly)
		Sunday	No workout			

A NEW HEALTHY YOU!
Workout Plan Schedule

DAY 65

Date	Week	Day	Exercise	Completed (x)	Weigh In	Workout Time
	1	Monday	No workout			
		Tuesday	Workout			30 minutes (Lightly)
		Wednesday	No workout			
		Thursday	Workout			30 minutes (Lightly)
		Friday	No workout			
		Saturday*	Workout			30 minutes (Lightly)
		Sunday	No workout			
	2	Monday	Workout			30 minutes (Lightly)
		Tuesday	No workout			
		Wednesday	Workout			30 minutes (Lightly)
		Thursday	No workout			
		Friday	Workout			30 minutes (Lightly)
		Saturday*	No workout			
		Sunday	Workout			30 minutes (Lightly)
	3	Monday	No workout			
		Tuesday	Workout			30 minutes (Lightly)
		Wednesday	No workout			
		Thursday	Workout			30 minutes (Lightly)
		Friday	No workout			
		Saturday*	Workout			30 minutes (Lightly)
		Sunday	No workout			

FINAL PAGE

CONGRATULATIONS ON THE NEW YOU!

This workbook has been made available on mobile devices via Adobe Digital Editions and DRM (Digital Rights Management).

NOTES

CONNECT WITH US

MAKING A DIFFERENCE IN THE LIVES OF MILLIONS, AROUND THE WORLD
Connect via Facebook Fan Page, YouTube and others by typing in **KYLA LATRICE MBA**

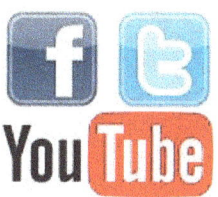

A WORKBOOK FOR AND WOMEN AND MEN

www.ingramcontent.com/pod-product-compliance
Lightning Source LLC
Chambersburg PA
CBHW080401030426
42334CB00024B/2953